Better Body
Basics

Mindset - Training - Nutrition - Recovery

John Wojciechowski, MS, CSCS

Table of Contents

"It is not the critic who counts; not the man who points out how the strong man stumbles, or where the doer of deeds could have done them better.

The credit belongs to the man who is actually in the arena, whose face is marred by dust and sweat and blood; who strives valiantly; who errs, who comes short again and again, because there is no effort without error and shortcoming; but who does actually strive to do the deeds; who knows great enthusiasms, the great devotions; who spends himself in a worthy cause; who at the best knows in the end the triumph of high achievement, and who at the worst, if he fails, at least fails while daring greatly, so that his place shall never be with those cold and timid souls who neither know victory nor defeat."

Theodore Roosevelt

Introduction

We've all heard the phrase, "You can't do everything."

While that phrase seems a bit pessimistic at first glance, there's some truth to the statement. People who try to do everything often lose focus on the things that really matter, and they ultimately end up accomplishing very little. People who fall into this trap work really hard, but perhaps they're not working as smart as they could be.

Working smarter means prioritizing your actions and spending your time and energy focused primarily on those activities from which you'll reap the greatest dividends.

The Pareto Principle is a principle borrowed from the business world, where it's been observed that often 80% of your results come from 20% of your efforts. The lesson here is to always stay focused on the important stuff that matters most and don't agonize over the small details.

This book is written in the spirit of this principle and will give you the tools to ensure that you are working smarter and taking the right steps on your own fitness journey.

This book is for those who are new to this lifestyle, who are attempting to transform themselves but don't know where to begin, and who are looking for an experienced perspective on the overall process. If you're completely new to the process, then you lack knowledge, experience, and perspective. Most of all, you probably lack confidence. My goal is that this book will help you understand all the pieces of the body transformation puzzle so you can feel confident in your approach and not waste time questioning your efforts.

This book is also for those of you who have been going at it for quite some time but keep getting stuck, sidetracked or distracted. Maybe you've been spinning your wheels, going months or even years without making progress, thinking you're doing the right thing but really not getting anywhere except frustrated. Maybe nagging little injuries keep rearing their ugly heads because you are doing or focusing on the wrong things. For you, this book will serve as a reminder to return to the basics and refocus your efforts on the things that matter most and actually drive progress.

An Experienced Perspective

Over the past 30 years, I have competed in various sports from gymnastics as a child to karate, wrestling, football and track and field in high school, earning all-state honors in football and track, winning an Eastern States Shot Put Championship, winning the coveted Penn Relays gold watch, and competing in the National Championships.

I received several scholarship offers and enjoyed regional success as a Division I track & field athlete, winning several team MVP honors, breaking school records, and competing in two more National Championships until I was sidelined by injuries.

As a young, fresh-faced college athlete, I was able to squat and deadlift over 600lbs and still perform a round-off, back-handspring back flip at a bodyweight of 260lbs. I had a good amount of raw talent, but I lacked a thorough understanding of the overall training process, which would have saved me an enormous amount of time, energy and frustration.

I've coached many athletes and adults over the years, from teens to retirees at track and field clinics, in large group training settings, small group training settings, boot camps and one-on-one helping people build muscle and lose fat.

I consider myself a journeyman, a jack of all trades; I've never specialized in any one pursuit for too long along the way. I've always had the unique ability to transform myself in pursuit of my particular goals, whatever they may have been at the time, always with successful results.

I admit I'm that annoying guy who shows up at your dinner

party with all sorts of dietary restrictions because I'm always experimenting on myself to see how various eating strategies affect how I look, feel and perform. Over the years, friends and family have joked that I've been somewhat of a chameleon, always gaining weight or losing weight for some reason or another, eating carbs this week and not eating carbs the next.

It's not that I've always approached my training properly. Quite the opposite: I've made plenty of mistakes along the way, but it's precisely those mistakes that have provided me the insight that you just can't acquire any other way. My goal is to share my perspective and experience with you so that you can learn what has worked for me and what I have seen work for my fellow coaches, friends and clients.

The Four Foundational Areas

In this book, I will discuss the principles and strategies of the four foundational areas that drive physical improvement—Mindset, Training, Nutrition, and Recovery—and I'll provide you with the perspective and understanding necessary for you to confidently approach your own transformation journey.

"If you want to be free,

Get to know your real self.

It has no form, no appearance,

No root, no basis, no abode,

but is lively and buoyant.

It responds with versatile facility,

but its function cannot be located.

Therefore, when you look for it,

you become further from it.

When you seek it,

You turn away from it all the more."

Linji

Chapter 1: Mindset

The first step in achieving your physical transformation is developing a strong and successful mindset, a set of mental skills that you can draw upon to help you reach your goals. Just like we need to develop our physical skills, we also need to practice and train these mental skills in order to grow stronger. Transformation is, first and foremost, a mental practice.

Cultivate Mindfulness

Success begins with the ability to focus on what you are doing in the here and now. We call this skill "mindfulness." Mindfulness is simply the practice of paying attention, remaining present, and developing our awareness. The depth to which we experience our lives is composed entirely of the totality of that which we are aware. We enrich our moment-to-moment experience of life by cultivating a deeper sense of mindfulness and increasing the sphere of our awareness. Our ability to operate from the present moment governs how we learn and is reflected in our level of personal productivity.

The ability to pay attention is a skill that can be practiced and developed. The simplest and most direct way to develop mindfulness is to set some time aside every day to sit undisturbed in a quiet place and simply practice paying attention. Become a witness to your thoughts without allowing yourself to become swept away by them. Allow your thoughts to arise and then fall away, always coming back to the present moment.

Most meditation practices emphasize placing your focus on the breath because our breath is always with us, and focusing on our breath helps anchor us in the present moment.

For more detailed information on meditation practice, I highly recommend the audio recording of *Alan Watts Teaches Meditation.*

Think Positive

Despite our best intentions, how many of us continue to engage in negative self-talk? Now that you're committed to cultivating mindfulness, you may be more aware than ever of just how negative and self-defeating some of your thoughts really are. The greater your awareness of these thoughts, the more able you will be to interrupt them and reframe them in a positive way.

If you want better answers, you have to ask yourself better questions. If you habitually ask yourself, "why do I always screw this up?," your mind probably comes up with plenty of reasons for you—even if they're untrue—and none of them are helpful or encouraging.

When you become aware of negative thoughts, quickly reframe them in a positive way in the form of positive statements or questions. Through this process, you put an end to self-destructive, negative thinking and begin to develop the habit of positive thinking.

Make a Commitment

Most people fail to see results because they lack commitment. You must be committed one hundred percent to achieving your goal. What you are committed to then becomes a priority in your life. You have to decide that you are going to do whatever it takes to achieve your own level of personal excellence. If you are wavering on your commitment, you will waver in your actions.

You have to be all-in. Full commitment is an absolute requirement. If you don't have that level of commitment, you will waver when the going gets tough.

Sure, you will stumble occasionally, but being totally committed means that you are committed to getting back up, dusting yourself off and continuing the journey no matter what obstacles you encounter.

When the Spanish conquistador Cortes landed in Veracruz in 1519, leading to the Spanish conquest of the Aztec Empire, he supposedly ordered his men to burn their own boats, leaving them no option for retreat. Cortes made sure that he and his men had no choice but to be entirely committed to the success of their endeavor. True or not, the story drives home the lesson of what it means to be 100% committed to success, leaving no option for failure.

What options for retreat or failure are you keeping for yourself? Don't undermine your own efforts. Burn those options for retreat now. Commit 100% and plan for success.

Connect With Your Deepest Why

Full commitment to your goals is virtually automatic when you can discover and stay connected to your deepest reasons for wanting to achieve them. Find the reason that is near and dear to your heart. This journey needs to be important to you, regardless of anyone else's support. If your "why" is strong enough, you will always find the "how."

Whatever It Takes

Life is not fair. We are all born into different socio-economic situations with different physical and mental aptitudes.

Some people are born with superb genetics that help them to become professional athletes, and others, not so much.

The truth is that some people will simply have to work harder or smarter, or even both, to make the same exact progress as the next guy. Never measure yourself against the progress someone else is making based on the work they are putting into it. Stay focused on your own efforts, and prepare to do whatever it takes to achieve your goals.

Give Up Magic Pills

When it comes to developing a plan for transformation, a lack of information is never the problem. All the information you'll ever need is already as close as the nearest Google search bar. The fact is that there's too much information, and most people are in a state of information overload.

The problem with having access to too much information is that trying to sift through all the half-truths, fads, and myths perpetuated by keyboard gurus is very difficult, and it can be nearly impossible to differentiate fact from fiction. If you don't already have a solid understanding of a particular topic, you will often fall for all sorts of deceptive marketing and advertising. These campaigns will try to sell you all sorts of programs, products, supplements and equipment you don't need with the promise to build slabs of muscle or shed unwanted pounds virtually overnight. These marketers are preying on most people's urge to look for a quick and easy path to their goals. I call this "Magic Pill Thinking."

You may understand this on an intellectual level, but somewhere deep inside, people still look for shortcuts to success, and there simply are no shortcuts. The desire to find that "brand new thing" that's going to catapult us toward our goals is an impulse that never quite leaves us, no matter how many times we've been around the block. This is why it's critically important to recognize those impulses when they arise and don't entertain them.

Set Goals

Now that you're committed one hundred percent to following through on your transformation, you need a method to direct your focus and track your progress. Goal setting is that method. Goals set our minds' intention, and our intentions govern our actions.

You likely have an idea in your head already of how you want to feel, what you want to look like, or how much you want to weigh after your transformation is complete. This vision is your long-term goal.

At the beginning, achieving your long-term goal can seem

like an insurmountable task. It may seem too far away to really wrap your brain around, maybe to the point that even contemplating your goal might feel discouraging. This is why we break down our long-term goal into a series of manageable short-term and intermediate goals that guide us toward achieving our long-term goal.

Your goals—daily, weekly, monthly, quarterly, yearly—should be reflective of each of the four foundational areas discussed in this book. For example, every day should have a mindset goal, a training goal, a nutrition goal, and a recovery goal.

These goals need to be written down and posted in a place where you will see them and be reminded of them on a daily basis. You must keep your goals constantly at the forefront of your mind. Post them on your refrigerator, on your bathroom mirror. Tape them to your laptop or the dashboard of your car, whatever it takes to keep you focused on success.

Your goals need to be specific, well-defined and non-contradictory. Your goals must also have a deadline, because deadlines create a sense of urgency. Your goals must be challenging to achieve but realistic in their timeframe.

Poorly Defined Goal: I want to get into better shape.

Well-Defined Goal: I'm going to lose 15 pounds over the

next three months by training four times per week at the group training center in my town and by following the nutrition plan that they lay out for me.

Some people like to keep their goals to themselves because they're afraid of being teased or of disappointing the people who support them if they fall short. Others like to share their goals with everyone they know to garner support and to create a greater sense of urgency to follow through. Pick the approach that best suits your personality.

Overall, you must remain focused on progress toward your goals, not perfection. You may fall short of your goals from time to time and have to readjust, but the true goal is making progress. Every step closer to your ultimate goal is still a step in the right direction. You just have to keep moving forward.

Keep a Journal

Goals, workouts, meals, sleep patterns, moods, energy levels, bodyweight, training ideas, and relevant thoughts should all be recorded in your training journal. Your training journal is your written master plan, and it will help guide the direction of your training. Over time you will notice emerging patterns: food choices that affect your mood or don't agree with your stomach, exercises that really help drive strength gains, how much sleep you really need to maximize your performance, or the time of day you have the most energy. If you're serious about your goals, keeping a journal is an absolute must for long term success.

Visualize Success

If you can see your goal in your mind's eye, you can achieve it. Now that you know how to calm your mind and center yourself through meditation, and you have a clearly defined goal, you can begin practicing visualization to help bring your success into greater focus. All successful people incorporate some sort of visualization into their routines. Visualizing yourself achieving the goals that you've set further solidifies the expectation that your goals can and will be achieved.

Imagine yourself with your ideal body. How do you look? How do you feel? Do you have more energy? Are you more confident? Do you feel more attractive? Create your own success story in your mind's eye. See it, and believe it.

Be Consistent

Once you have your goals set, you need to practice and develop the patience and discipline to achieve them, and then you must pursue them with consistency. Consistency is your key to making progress. Your commitment must be 24/7, not a part-time endeavor. Like Vince Lombardi stated, "Winning is an all-the-time thing." Every meal, every good night's sleep, every workout builds on the previous one, and so on. Consistency builds momentum. It's the snowball effect, and it's important both physically and psychologically. This is how real progress happens, slowly and consistently over time.

A mason who starts building a brick wall lays brick on top of brick, day after day, and the wall gets higher and higher. If that mason disappears for two weeks and comes back to start working again, the wall will be the same height that he left it, and he can continue where he left off. This means the mason can work on the wall whenever he feels like it and still see great progress over the course of time. This is the way some people think that training works, and they're wrong.

Yes, every successful day of following your eating strategy or training program adds another brick to the wall, but the difference between us and the mason is that bricks fall back off the wall when we train too infrequently, stuff our faces too often, or don't take the proper steps to recover sufficiently in between our training sessions. We must be consistent.

Be Patient

If you do the right things consistently, you must have the patience to trust the process. Patience is a virtue, and you absolutely need it in order to stay the course and enjoy the journey. There are no overnight successes when it comes to achieving something truly worth achieving.

Real transformation is a marathon, not a sprint. Progress seems to happen slowly because most people want overnight results. You can make amazing changes over the course of several weeks and even more over several months, but it requires patience to stick it out.

Sure, your goal might be to lose 10 pounds, but you have to focus on pound number one, then pound number two, and so on. The same goes for the person who just benched 225 pounds, and now they have their sights set on 315. You first have to get to 230, then 235, and so on.

A lack of patience is where people fall prey to the magic pill mindset. When this happens, people change training programs and diets as often as they change their socks, and those are the people that see lackluster results, if any.

Be Disciplined

To operate with a sense of discipline is to recognize that the actions you choose to take at any particular moment are part of a larger plan to bring you closer to your goals. You realize, when you're disciplined, that in order to reach your goal, your actions must be consistent with the purpose of your plan, regardless of your present level of motivation or current feelings. Discipline is choosing between what you want now and what you want most.

You must have the self-discipline to execute the plan you are committed to. You cannot allow yourself to be dissuaded by people and circumstances. A person who exhibits great discipline doesn't fall to the level of doing what he wants to do for immediate gratification. He elevates himself to the level of doing what he needs to do to move closer to his vision of success.

Stay Focused

Where your focus goes, energy flows. You must approach your workouts with a focused determination. This doesn't mean that you can't have fun in the gym, but the fun comes second to the primary goal, which is getting your work done. How heavy or light a weight feels when you try to lift it depends in part on your ability to focus on the task at hand.

If you are maintaining an ongoing conversation with your workout partner while you are actually performing the various exercises, you are, by definition, not focused 100% on what you are doing, and, therefore, you are not working very hard.

You must learn to practice selective attention and develop your ability to move from a broad focus of attention to a narrow focus of attention during your work sets. Along with the development of greater focus will come the ability to control the level of energy that you can bring to your training.

We call this energy your "state of arousal." Extremely high levels of arousal are typically witnessed in competition environments. You can imagine watching a powerlifter or a shot putter getting psyched up before an attempt. Their level of arousal is generally extremely high. I'm not suggesting you need to get all worked up before every set of squats like it's a matter of life and death, but you need to focus hard and give your best effort during your training sessions for maximum results.

No Excuses

The list of excuses that I've heard people make over the years about why they can't make it to the gym or why they're not making progress with their current training program is astonishingly long. People blame their jobs, spouses, kids, physicians, personal trainers, real or imagined aches and pains, you name it. But the responsibility for your success and failure always lies squarely on your shoulders alone and nobody else's. Responsibility is not something your trainer can give to you; it's something you have to take for yourself and own.

Good Enough is Not Good Enough

If you want to be successful, you need to hold yourself to the strictest of standards, even when others don't, and even when nobody is looking. If the task is to sprint 100 yards, then 99 yards is not good enough. If the task is to bear crawl all the way to the wall, then walking the last 10 feet before you touch the wall is not good enough.

Before you misunderstand me, I'm not talking about someone who lacks the physical ability to perform a certain task or is otherwise truly giving 100%. I'm talking about those who have not yet developed that certain sense of honesty with themselves that drives them to do things the right way every time when they are perfectly capable.

How you do anything is how you do everything, and cutting corners while telling yourself "that's good enough" will bleed into every other area of your life. Champions do not cut corners, and you are the champion of your own life.

Ignore the Haters

Success will attract haters. Some people have a really hard time supporting other people's efforts to achieve a level of personal excellence that they themselves are unwilling to commit to and work toward. Some people will discourage you or outright mock you and the goals you have set for yourself. Some of your friends, co-workers, and even closest family members will not appreciate you rocking the boat and pursuing a healthier lifestyle because it sheds a light on their own bad habits. You will need to grow a thick skin and stick to your guns.

Don't ever allow others to drag you down to their level. Don't ever change course to save other people's feelings. Like the Marianne Williamson quote says, "Your playing small does not serve the world."

"No man has the right to be an amateur in the matter of physical training. It is a shame for a man to grow old without ever seeing the beauty and strength of which his body is capable."

Socrates

Chapter 2: Training

Training vs. Exercise

Before we discuss the types of training we need to do to maximize progress, we have to make a distinction between training and exercise.

Too many people go to the gym and wander from machine to machine, just doing what feels good to them on any given day, with no particular plan for the day and no thought as to how their workout fits into a larger plan to move them toward their goals. This is just exercise, and you must train to gain.

Training is planned, organized, progressive, goal-oriented activity designed to introduce a specific stimulus to the body to encourage a specific positive adaptation. Training has purpose. What most people call "exercise" generally lacks this type of organized approach.

Training means having a plan for every workout. Even if your plan does not specifically outline the sets and reps you are planning to do, you must be clear on your overall intent for the workout before you walk through the gym door. You need to know what you are aiming to accomplish and how it fits into the bigger picture.

Furthermore, the goal-oriented nature of training means it also carries with it the risk of failure. Cultivating the perseverance to deal with this added stress builds character and develops mental toughness. Casual exercise lacks this long-term mental and emotional commitment.

Gym Etiquette

Let's do a quick review of proper gym etiquette. Most of this will, hopefully, be common sense. A gym is a community of like-minded people, so you must demonstrate respect for your community to be a successful member.

Always be courteous and work on the assumption that the other people sharing the gym space with you are there to work hard too, not to socialize. There's a difference between being polite and enjoying some small talk between sets versus being that completely unfocused person who seems completely disconnected from the task at hand and becomes a distraction to everyone around them.

Everyone is at the gym to work hard, and hard work requires concentration, so respect people's personal space and don't do anything that might break their concentration during the workout. Don't load or unload plates onto racks while others are using them, don't walk between someone and their reflection if they are using a mirror to check their form during a set, and don't ever try to talk to someone while they are performing a set, even if it's only to ask a question. Never, ever try to steal a person's attention from the work they are performing.

When you use something, put it back where it belongs so the next person can easily find it. Never leave a loaded barbell on the floor or in the rack for someone else to deal with. Strip the bar, and put the plates back where they belong.

Unless you absolutely require your cell phone for emergency purposes, do yourself and everyone around you a favor and leave it in your locker or in your car. Give yourself the best opportunity for success by being unreachable for an hour so you can focus on yourself.

This is just a partial list, so use common sense. A little self-awareness goes a long way. Learning and following proper gym etiquette shows respect for the art of training, the gym, and the other members.

Don't Neglect Your Warm-Up

A proper warm-up serves many purposes. It increases your core temperature, increases respiration and blood flow, delivering oxygen to tissues, and wakes up your central nervous system. Warming up also gives you an opportunity to be sure that you can comfortably move through the ranges of motion that will be required by your workout by "checking-in" with your body to see if you have any especially tight areas or strange sensations that you hadn't been previously aware of.

Focus on dynamic movements and light stretching as opposed to excessively long bouts of static stretching prior to training. Long periods of static stretching immediately prior to training have been shown to interfere with muscle force production.

Remember, your warm-up is as much for your mind as it is for your body. It provides a transitionary period to let go of whatever you had been previously focused on, like work or family issues. It gets you re-focused on your goals for this training session and the effort you're about to put forth.

In addition to your general warm-up, every major exercise deserves its own specific warm-up. Always start with an empty bar and work up in weight to your working sets in moderate increments. Treat these warm-up sets with the same attention and focus on technique as your heaviest sets. These lighter, warm-up sets prepare your body and mind for your heavier sets and provide the opportunity to further develop your technique. Strength is not just about muscle, strength is a skill that requires practice.

Resistance Training

Resistance training can be defined as exerting muscular force against an external resistance for the purpose of developing strength and increasing muscle tissue size (hypertrophy). If your goal is to get big and strong, then hitting the weights is obviously your main focus. However, any time you're looking to lose bodyfat through a combination of diet and increased activity, you need to incorporate resistance training into your routine as well. Reducing calories and doing lots of cardio without resistance training increases the risk of muscle tissue loss and we want to ensure that weight loss comes from fat stores. In plain English, you have to give your body a reason why it should continue to invest so much of its own energy keeping so much muscle tissue hanging around. If you don't use it, you will eventually lose it.

What are Muscles, and How Do They Work?

The type of muscle we are talking about here is skeletal muscle tissue as opposed to cardiac muscle (heart muscle) or smooth muscle found in organs, which are not under voluntary control. Skeletal muscle like your biceps, for example, is comprised of strands of fasciculi, which are bundles of single muscle fibers. Each muscle fiber is a bundle of myofibrils, which are comprised of actin and myosin filaments. These filaments are arranged longitudinally in segments called sarcomeres, which are the smallest contractile units of skeletal muscle. During muscle contraction, the actin filaments slide over the myosin filaments, and this is known as the sliding filament theory of muscle contraction.

There are three basic muscle fiber types: slow-twitch Type I, fast-twitch Type IIa, and fast-twitch Type IIb. As the names imply, slow-twitch fibers develop force slowly but fatigue more slowly as well, while fast-twitch fibers develop force quickly but also fatigue more quickly. Different skeletal muscles contain different ratios of these fibers, and this goes for people, overall, as well.

All else being equal, a muscle with a larger cross sectional area is a stronger muscle. This is why we still train to increase muscle size even if strength is our primary goal.

Why Train for Strength?

Physical strength is the foundation for all other physical qualities, and resistance training is the most efficient way to increase physical strength and build muscle mass. Resistance training also strengthens connective tissue, increases bone density, improves joint mobility, and even improves cardiovascular fitness. No other form of training can claim all of these benefits.

All human movements can be more or less condensed into variations or combinations of what Holistic Health Practitioner Paul Check calls the 7 primal movement patterns: bending, squatting, pushing, pulling, twisting, lunging, and gait (walking/running). A well-rounded strength training program will include variations of these basic movement patterns under load and through the full range of motion.

Another important point that cannot be overstated is that the amount of physical strength and muscle tissue that you can develop and maintain heading into your older years is directly proportional to the quality of life you will enjoy at that age. We should all think of regular training as banking strength and muscle that we can draw upon later in life when our very lives may depend on our ability to recover from a fall, bounce back from a disease, or just continue to live independently.

Barbells are for Everyone

When it comes to resistance training, barbells are king. If you are otherwise healthy and capable, then movements like the barbell squat, barbell bench, barbell deadlift, and standing barbell press should make up the core of your resistance training program because these barbell exercises recruit the greatest number of muscles around the greatest number of joints in the body. These exercises help your muscles to work in coordination with one another to generate the greatest amount of force required to stabilize and move the heaviest loads possible. These barbell exercises disrupt your body's homeostasis to the greatest degree to provide the best possible stimulus for gaining strength and building muscle.

Dumbbells, machines, and body weight exercises all play a supporting role, but your primary barbell movements take center stage. Of course, not everyone has the strength, skill, coordination or mobility to climb under a loaded barbell their first day at the gym. There are logical regressions and progressions to these movements that a good coach will prescribe that are appropriate to your current level of development.

It's not that you absolutely must train with barbells in order to make progress, but if you want to maximize your progress, make the most efficient use of your time and effort, and reach as close to your physical potential as possible, then why wouldn't you?

Even if you are not using barbells, you should always prioritize multi-joint exercises over single joint exercises in your workout because of their ability to provide a greater stimulus to the body for overall strength and muscle gains.

Proper Form

Always perform your repetitions with proper form and under control. Never sacrifice proper form to add weight to the bar or to get extra reps. In the long run, this is counter-productive and can lead to injury. You must practice proper form from the moment you begin your warm-up on an exercise. You want to treat the light weights with the same focus and respect that you treat the heavy weights. Your technical execution of the lift should look the same whether you are benching the bar or attempting a new personal best.

Take a Deep Breath

How you breathe is critical to your success in the weight room. On your big barbell lifts, you want to take a deep belly breath and brace your core before each repetition. Inhale deeply, and hold your breath during the eccentric (lowering or negative) portion of the lift and during the initial phase of the concentric (upward or positive) portion of the lift until you know you've got the rep. Repeat this for all your reps.

Holding your breath and bracing in this way is also known as the Valsalva maneuver and involves exhaling against a closed glottis. This increases your intra-abdominal and intrathoracic pressures, helping to stabilize your spine and create greater stability for lifting heavier weights, as well as reducing the risk of injury.

Rest Periods

Rest periods between sets and exercises for resistance training can vary somewhat greatly based on what type of training stimulus you are going for, but generally you are shooting for adequate recovery between sets until you feel like you're ready to go hard again. For this reason, rest periods typically fall somewhere in the 1 to 3 minute range depending on the exercise and intensity level.

Building Muscle While Losing Fat

If your goal is fat loss, this is not the time for backing off on your resistance training. This is precisely the time you need to fight for every ounce of muscle on your body. You must continue to train like an animal in the weight room simply to prevent muscle loss as a consequence of calorie restriction. Whether you are following a fat loss protocol or not, at a minimum you are always in a battle with Father Time, so you must always keep your foot on the gas.

Building muscle and losing fat at the same time is certainly possible, especially for the new trainee. However, the longer you have been training, the more difficult it becomes. Typically, it is much easier to maintain existing muscle mass while losing body fat than to add new muscle. This is why most approaches to body transformation include alternating periods of bulking and cutting.

Muscle is gained much more easily in an environment where calories are plentiful. The goal in a bulking phase is to eat just enough over your maintenance calories to gain muscle while minimizing fat gain.

Fat loss is best achieved in a calorie restrictive environment, so the goal in your cutting phase is to lose as much body fat as possible while maintaining your muscle.

Muscle tissue is like having your own personal calorie furnace. Gaining muscle tissue increases the amount of calories you burn every day just to maintain your bodyweight, making it easier to lose fat. A loss of muscle tissue lowers your metabolism and makes it more difficult to lose fat.

The biggest mistake I see people make with their approach to resistance training while "on a diet" is that they convince themselves that they can't get stronger or gain muscle while also losing body fat, or they simply decide that they're going to lose the weight first and then start resistance training.

Falling into this trap, they lighten their weights, reduce their training focus and intensity, and basically allow themselves to go into some sort of cruise control mode in the weight room. This approach can result in unwanted and counter-productive muscle loss. Of course the worst decision you can make is to not resistance train at all.

Cardiovascular Training

Cardiovascular training is generally done for several different reasons: to improve or maintain basic cardiovascular health, to improve the energy demands for a particular sport, or to use it as a tool to burn additional calories to further facilitate fat loss.

Cardiovascular exercise is a great tool for fat loss, but too often people misunderstand it and abuse it in their efforts to shed pounds. Some people see endless hours on the treadmill as another magic pill that's going to strip off their body fat in record time, and that's not the best approach.

Cardiovascular exercise generally falls into two categories: steady-state cardio and interval training. The specific type of interval training that we'll be discussing here is known as high-intensity interval training (HIIT).

Before we discuss these two types of cardio, let's review how our bodies create and utilize energy.

Energy Systems

Adenosine Triphosphate (ATP) is our body's energy currency, and our body draws from a collective pool of ATP for all of its energy needs.

Our muscle cells only store ATP in limited amounts, so ATP constantly needs to be replenished through three different pathways or energy systems that each work to greater or lesser degrees depending on the intensity and duration of our activity.

The Phosphagen System provides ATP from stored creatine phosphate in skeletal muscle for high-intensity, short duration activities lasting up to about 10 seconds (a 100-meter sprint, for example). This system does not require oxygen, nor does it produce lactate (commonly referred to as lactic acid). It is the energy system used at the very beginning of all activity.

The Glycolytic System provides ATP from the breakdown of carbohydrates from stored muscle glycogen and blood glucose for moderate to high intensity activity lasting up to a few minutes (an 800-meter run). This system does not require oxygen, either, but it does produce lactate, which causes that feeling of burning in your muscles.

The Oxidative System provides ATP from the breakdown

41

of carbohydrates and fats while your body is at rest and for low intensity, long duration activity (such as a 5K run). This system requires oxygen and is the most complex of the three energy systems, producing the most ATP. This system is also known as the Aerobic System, and it's why cardio classes became known as "Aerobics."

Steady-State Cardio

Steady-state cardio generally refers to an exercise that elevates your heart rate to a moderate range and maintains your heart rate in that range for the duration of your workout. The primary energy system being used here would be the Oxidative System.

Walking, jogging, or bike riding are popular options for steady-state cardio. It burns extra calories, and it is a good starting point for some people who are new to exercise.

The downside to steady state cardio is that, by definition, you are working at a low intensity and not burning a whole lot of calories or fat. Also, your body adapts to this low-intensity work rather quickly, becoming more efficient at utilizing its energy sources, so over time your body burns fewer calories for the same amount of work. You can see how this can be incredibly frustrating for someone looking to lose body fat.

High-Intensity Interval Training

Alternating between short periods of high-intensity effort and short periods of low-intensity effort or rest is known as high-intensity interval training. A simple example of this would be sprinting 40 yards, walking back to the starting line, immediately sprinting again, and repeating for a specific number of rounds depending on your current level of conditioning.

HIIT allows you to burn more calories in a shorter amount of time while improving the performance of all three energy systems at the same time. The reverse is not true, however. Spending all your time performing steady state cardio does not improve the performance of your Phosphagen or Glycolytic systems.

Since HIIT improves the performance of all three energy systems, you'll also have more gas in the weight room to push yourself harder and complete more work.

HIIT also induces a metabolic condition known as "Excess Post-Exercise Oxygen Consumption" or EPOC.

EPOC allows your body to burn calories at a higher rate for many hours following your workout as your body consumes more oxygen while seeking to restore itself to its pre-workout level of homeostasis. Sometimes people refer to this as the "after burn" effect.

It should be clear by now that several HIIT sessions per week is a perfect complement to your resistance training for improving your overall conditioning, cardiovascular health, and body composition. Just keep in mind that HIIT is an intense activity that needs to be programmed wisely so as to not overload your ability to recover. If you are an athlete, the work-to-rest ratios of your HIIT sessions should mirror the work-to-rest ratios of your sport.

People often ask when the perfect time is to perform their HIIT workouts. The simple answer is whenever it fits your schedule and you can get it done. The only time I would recommend *not* performing your HIIT training is directly before your resistance training. Successful resistance training depends on your ability to lift the heaviest loads you are able to, so you don't want to begin your resistance training workout already fatigued.

Mobility and Flexibility

Some mobility and flexibility work should be included in everyone's routine, especially as we grow older. Maintaining normal range of movement around our joints is necessary to create the stability required to properly perform movements in the weight room without pain or discomfort, and it also helps to reduce the risk of injury.

Consider the amount of energy your body invests in maintaining the tension you experience in the various parts of your body. Imagine the amount of energy your system can reclaim by relaxing these areas through mobility and flexibility practice and improved postural alignment.

Give Yoga a Try

Yoga is a movement practice that was developed thousands of years ago to help prepare a person's body and mind for meditation practice. Yoga is a general term that encompasses many different styles of practice, which all differ in purpose and difficulty.

Yoga is an excellent choice for improving mobility and flexibility in an organized and progressive manner as well as greatly helping to improve your mind-muscle connection and breathing skills. Yoga also calms the mind and reduces stress.

Dealing with Injuries

Sorry to hit you with the obvious, but at some point you are probably going to experience an injury. This is just a part of the game. Injuries come in different magnitudes, from strains and muscle pulls to tears that require surgical re-attachment. In all cases, the worst thing that you can do is to completely stop training when you're injured.

My first word of advice is to take full responsibility for your own rehabilitation, and this starts with education. At the end of the day, it's your body and your responsibility. Learn all you can about your injury, types of rehab, types of surgeries (if applicable), how others have successfully rehabbed their injuries, etc. Don't just simply fall in line with whatever your doctor tells you because you happen to like and trust them or, worse, because you're too lazy to investigate your options for yourself. Doctors are notoriously conservative in their guidance in order to avoid litigation.

I have learned for myself that movement is healing. The more blood I can circulate through and around an injured area, the faster it heals. Training around an injury also keeps you fully engaged in the training process and keeps you showing up, working hard, and eating right.

I choose not to take anti-inflammatory meds or to ice injured areas so as to not interfere with the lymphatic system's natural inflammatory response to injury. I choose instead to use movement to improve circulation and avoid excessive swelling. This is not medical advice. I can only share with you what I have found to work best for myself.

When I tore my ACL years ago, I followed my doctor's orders to the letter. I never did any more work than was prescribed, and I attended every rehabilitation session doing exactly as they told me. To this day, I have not regained complete range of motion of my left knee, and it's because I didn't have the wherewithal to take responsibility for my own rehab.

When I tore my biceps, it was a different story. I was intent on trusting myself and my instincts, using common sense and pain as a guide. Before my surgery, I watched a video of the surgery I was going to have being performed so I had an excellent idea of exactly what was going to happen. I reached out to other athletes who had torn their biceps and asked questions. I developed my own timeline and goals for my own rehabilitation based on my own research. Beginning the day after surgery, I would perform several of my own rehab sessions throughout the day, removing my brace and beginning the process of flexing and extending my arm to the smallest degree. I would also allow my arm to hang without support, dealing with the discomfort as gravity gently stretched my arm slowly toward extension.

I knew I would not be able to hold a regular barbell on my back to squat or hold a bar to deadlift for some time after my surgery, so I purchased something called a safety squat bar that incorporates a padded yoke, allowing this bar to sit fairly balanced on your shoulders requiring only one good arm to hold it in place. Within a day or two after my surgery, I was using my safety squat bar for squats, good mornings, shrugs, and anything else I could think of.

Taking control of my own rehab allowed me to physically and mentally stay in the game and advance much faster than strictly following doctor's orders would have allowed. Of course, I'm not recommending you ignore your doctor. I'm simply sharing these stories to illustrate the importance of educating yourself and not just blindly following what medical professionals may recommend to you.

The Value of a Good Coach

Lots of people shy away from going to the gym because it conjures up images of muscle-bound men in tank tops, sweating and grunting while throwing around heavy barbells. Quite frankly, this image can be very intimidating to the uninitiated. Even if you can manage the confidence to walk through the doors of your local gym, where do you even start? How do you know what exercises to do? How many exercises do you do, and in what order do you do them, and for how many sets and reps, and with what weight?

Never follow some random non-specific training routine

you found in some magazine article about some celebrity's training routine, claiming to be the Holy Grail for getting huge and ripped or slim and sexy. The process of developing a training plan can seem very confusing and intimidating, which is why it is extremely important to seek out the advice of an experienced and knowledgeable coach. Without the proper guidance, most people lack the confidence to truly push themselves and put forth the effort required to make progress.

Having the right coach can literally save you years of learning through trial and error. A good coach will keep you progressing at the appropriate speed, reinforce good technique, prevent you from developing bad habits, keep you from making bad decisions that may lead to injury, and provide accountability. A coach will also provide guidance on developing the proper mindset and optimizing your nutrition and recovery.

Principles That Govern Training Progress

Finding and working with a knowledgeable coach doesn't nullify what I said earlier about you having ultimate responsibility for your own success. Therefore, it's important to have a basic understanding of the rules of the game before you get started.

Stimulus-Recovery-Adaptation (SRA)

SRA is the training principle that describes the process through which we introduce a stimulus to the body in the form of a training session or a series of training sessions, recover, and adapt in a positive way.

Let's say we introduce a stimulus to the body in the form of a lower-body resistance-training session. Initially, there is a short period of time after our training session where our capabilities are diminished. However, after some additional recovery time, our body grows a little stronger than we were before. This is the window of opportunity to train again.

The idea is that you need to perform enough hard work over a given period of time that it provides a great enough stimulus for the body to adapt without performing too much work so that your body can't recover from it and, therefore, can't positively adapt to it. This is why consistency is so important. If too much time passes before the next round of stimulus, our bodies will have lost some or all of the gains that we previously made, and we'll be starting from scratch again. On the other hand, if we continue to bombard ourselves with workout after workout, and we don't allow for enough recovery to take place, then we can quickly burn ourselves out or even get injured.

We want to approach, but not step over, the line here. Due to individual differences, this line is different for everyone. The goal here is to train optimally, not maximally.

Large muscle groups like legs and the back require longer periods of recovery because of the heavier loads used, as compared to smaller muscles like your biceps. Always use common sense; if you're feeling particularly beat up, then you probably need some more rest. Train hard, but always err on the side of caution. We're in this for the long haul, so sometimes it's better to live to fight another day than to keep grinding yourself down.

The S.A.I.D. Principle

S.A.I.D. stands for Specific Adaptation to Imposed Demands, and it simply means that our bodies adapt in a very specific way to the demands that we place upon it. Therefore, the stimulus we provide must be specific to the adaptation we are looking for. This should be a fairly obvious principle, but it gets overlooked quite often.

If you want to squat 500 pounds, then you need to squat heavy and often. All the lunges and leg extensions in the world won't get you there. For best results, you must practice the way you want to play.

Volume-Intensity-Frequency

The dose of specific stimulus that we provide to the body must be measured and balanced so it can be programmed and managed properly. We do this by controlling the volume, intensity, and frequency of the work we perform. There is an inverse relationship amongst all three variables for a given recovery ability, so an immediate increase in one requires the maintenance or decrease of the others.

Volume refers to the total amount of work performed. For lifters, it can be measured in total pounds by multiplying your sets times reps times weight. Only count your heavy work sets in this total. Lighter warm-up sets generally are not of a sufficient intensity level to have any impact on your ability to recover.

Intensity doesn't refer to the effort someone puts forth, per se, in the way we would say, "That guy trains with intensity!"

For lifters, intensity refers to the amount of resistance being used (mass of the barbell) in reference to your one rep maximum (1RM) and therefore is represented as a percentage of your 1RM. If your best squat is 300 pounds for one rep, then 150 pounds is 50% of 1RM and, thus, a fairly low intensity. A squat of 270 pounds, however, is 90% of 1RM and, thus, a very high intensity.

Most people will benefit the most from spending a majority of their training time using moderately heavy loads in the 5-10 rep range because that produces the best stimulus for a combination of strength and muscle gain. A moderately heavy load is generally in the range of 70%-85% of 1RM.

Frequency refers to the number of training sessions performed over a given period of time, or the number of times you perform a particular exercise over a given period.

Progressive Overload

The stimulus that you provide your body must progressively increase over the course of time in order for you to make continued progress. Those who perform the same exercises in the same order with the same weights for the same sets and reps with the same rest periods week after week will quickly cease to make progress. You must continue to challenge yourself in one way or another week after week, month after month, to make continued progress. A well-designed program will provide the framework to make this happen and prevent stall-outs.

Variety

Incorporating a reasonable variety of exercises in your training is a great way to keep things interesting and present new challenges. However, exercise variety in and of itself is not a driving force for continued progress. The point here is that there is a balance to be struck between specificity and variety depending on your goals.

K.I.S.S.

There is beauty in simplicity. I have always found it best to keep your approach simple and focused on the basics for best results. A simple and well-executed approach to your training is always better than an overly complex approach that is difficult to implement, track, and manage. Don't try to be too clever with your approach. You can't possibly account for every single variable that may affect your performance on any given day.

Remember, we're focused on making progress, and there will never be such a thing as a perfect plan. Complexity is the enemy of execution. Like George Patton once said, "A good plan violently executed now is better than a perfect plan executed next week."

Riding the Rollercoaster

Not every single workout is going to be better than the last; nobody's progress is completely linear. You're going to have good days and bad days, just as in life itself. Training requires you to be flexible and adapt your expectations on any given day.

Like Mike Tyson said, "Everybody has a plan until they get punched in the face." Sometimes life punches you in the face, and your training sessions are a real struggle. Sometimes you feel like a superhero, like you can take on the world. Both of these extremes can be expected every so often. Don't curse the crappy days; just take them in stride. And don't hold your breath for the superhero days; they'll show up every now and again when you least expect it.

Most of the time, however, you should just feel pretty good. When you are consistently stringing together lots of "pretty good" days, you know your training is on the right track.

Sometimes when you find yourself in a good rhythm making consistent progress week after week, it can almost seem too easy. You will be tempted to tinker with your current program to try and accelerate the progress you are already making…don't do this. Whatever you are currently doing is obviously working, so don't fix it if it ain't broken. More is not always better. Progress is progress…and slow and steady progress is certainly better than no progress at all. If your current plan is working, stick to it.

Remember that gaining strength and building muscle is a life-long pursuit. It's a marathon, not a sprint. The true practice is becoming increasingly in-tune with your body's needs and discovering what works best for you. What works best for you today may change six months from now. Keep learning and listening to your body, and stay flexible in your approach.

Get Comfortable Being Uncomfortable

Make no mistake, effective training will not always be "fun" in the way that we typically define the word. There will be days that you just need to get the work done regardless of how you feel about it. Training is not a pursuit of the ego, so we are not seeking pleasure or the avoidance of pain or discomfort. We are training for something greater than immediate gratification.

The lessons we learn about ourselves and the physical improvements that we realize over months and years of hard, consistent training are so fulfilling that we develop the will-ingness to endure the pain and discomfort of intense phys-ical effort. Remember, if it doesn't challenge you, it doesn't change you.

"Let food be thy medicine,

and medicine be thy food."

Hippocrates

Chapter 3: Nutrition

We literally are what we eat. I know we've all heard of that before, but take a moment to really consider that statement. The way our bodies look, the way we feel, the particular health issues we may or may not be facing are all rooted primarily in the quality of our nutrition. Read that one more time, because this point can't be overstated. You can train as hard and as long as you want, but if you are consuming an excess of nutritionally hollow processed foods, or you are chronically dehydrated, your health will suffer, and you will never look and perform anywhere near your best.

The First Step

The main focus of any effective nutrition plan—and my recommendation for the first thing you should do as you develop a transformation plan—is to always focus on improving the quality of your food by eating a variety of whole, natural, unprocessed foods. At the same time, work to ensure full hydration and the consumption of all of the essential proteins, fats, vitamins and minerals.

There are many types of diets out there that go by all sorts of catchy names, but I have found that the most effective eating strategies share the same common principles: reduction of excess processed carbohydrates (especially simple sugars), adequate high-quality protein intake to support muscle growth, adequate healthy fat intake, and an emphasis on whole, natural, unprocessed food sources.

Stay Hydrated

One of the quickest and easiest steps you can take to improve your performance and overall health is to ensure you are drinking enough water every day. The general minimum recommendation is about half of your bodyweight in ounces per day, so a 200lb man should aim for 100 ounces of water per day. How much water you actually need is determined by many different factors that include the climate where you live and your activity level. If you are waiting to drink water until you feel thirsty, then you are not fully hydrated.

Good and Bad Foods

There are no good foods or bad foods, per se. Food is completely neutral. It has no agenda. The basics of what we need for survival are, in the most basic terms, water, essential amino acids, essential fatty acids, and the essential vitamins and minerals. Everything else can simply be seen as being either supportive or not supportive of your transformation goals.

Of course there are foods we can probably all agree on that are "bad" in a sense, but I emphasize this point primarily to combat magic pill thinkers who read the fad diet advice in magazines who will run out to the supermarket and stock their refrigerator with this fruit or that yogurt because some article in a magazine said it was "good" for them or would help "burn belly fat" or some other such nonsense. This is an extremely narrow view of nutrition, and you must seek to develop a basic understanding of the bigger picture.

Your Starting Point

I always recommend that you start where you are. By that, I mean that you should simply accept where you are right now and make small changes from there. The way you look and feel at this very moment is the perfect reflection of your existing lifestyle and habits. Even if you are far from looking and feeling the way you want, you can still consider your nutrition and training routine already a success, because you are getting perfect results based on your current behavior.

If you're not happy with where you are, the good news is that you can easily change your results by changing your actions. This process is not outside of your control.

A Strategy That Works

In order for your new eating strategy to be a success, it needs to be easy to implement and to stick to. Ease of compliance is the most important factor in developing a nutrition plan that will be successful. This is why I recommend a habits based approach, encouraging people to start slowly with small, manageable changes and build momentum from there I promise you, these small changes will add up over time.

The most common approach to dieting is usually to scrap everything you've been doing up until this very moment in order to "put yourself" on a diet. This usually means a pretty dramatic change in what you've been eating, along with a bunch of other unrealistic sweeping changes in your routine, such as going from zero days of exercise to daily trips to the gym.

This is why most people are fearful of dieting and exercise and end up failing over and over again. It's too much too soon. It takes you too far outside your comfort zone, and it makes you feel overwhelmed. This is why I always emphasize ease of compliance. The best laid plans don't mean anything if you don't follow through with them.

The truth is that your body can only burn fat and/or synthesize new muscle tissue so quickly. There's simply no advantage to be gained by making dramatic sweeping changes to your existing diet and exercise plan unless, of course, you're directed to do so by a physician due to medical reasons.

One Thing at a Time

You can start by eliminating sugar from your diet by swapping out regular soda for a diet soda. Or you could try reducing the portion size of just one of your meals per day. These are pretty small changes, but they will build the mindfulness and habits necessary to build upon going forward. Once you are already moving in the right direction, you simply have to be patient and consistent, and you have to allow things to happen.

There's no shortcut to the process. Looking for a shortcut is magic pill thinking. You didn't just wake up this morning 20 pounds overweight, so those 20 pounds are not going to come off overnight, either. Be consistent, and be patient.

Dieting Misconceptions

There are several popular misconceptions about dieting that I'd like to cover. First of all, lots of people go on a diet only when they are looking to shed some pounds. Most people see dieting as a temporary state, a particular period of time during which they're going to achieve some weight loss goal. After that period is over, they think they are going to return to their normal habits and maintain their new body. This perspective on dieting is deeply flawed because it's precisely your normal habits that created this need to lose weight. Because of that, dieting should not be approached as something you're going to stop as soon as you lose the weight. Real transformation is a permanent lifestyle change, not a temporary fix.

Lots of people also believe that you can eat whatever you want just because you exercise. Nobody would love for this to be true more than me, but, unfortunately, it's not. Exercising does not give you license to stop paying attention to nutrition without consequences. Often, people use their training as a convenient excuse to use food as a reward, and that's a dangerous game.

You should also always keep in mind that there's no magic food. This goes along with everything I've already said about magic pill thinking and the fact that foods are neither good nor bad. Foods either serve a purpose to you nutritionally by supporting your performance and body composition goals, or they don't. It's that simple.

Understand, too, that not all calories are created equal. A 2,000-calorie diet composed of meats and veggies has a vastly different effect on your body than a 2,000-calorie diet composed of soda and potato chips.

Calories Explained

One kilocalorie is the amount of energy required to raise the temperature of one liter of water by one degree Celsius at sea level. For nutrition purposes and nutrition labeling, we commonly refer to kilocalories as simply calories. It's the way we measure the energy we derive from food. There are 3,500 calories in a pound, meaning that to reduce your body weight by one pound in one week, you need to create a weekly caloric deficit of 3,500 calories through diet and exercise.

The Role of Macronutrients

There are three macronutrients found in food: protein, fat, and carbohydrates.

Protein

We primarily associate protein with its role in muscle repair and growth, but protein serves many different functions in the body, from maintenance of healthy cell structure to hormonal regulation. Protein is composed of twenty-two building blocks called "amino acids." Thirteen of these amino acids can be synthesized in the body, but the other nine are considered essential amino acids and must be consumed in our diet.

Protein in food contains four calories per gram. When you're deciding how much protein you need in your diet, shoot for approximately .8 grams of protein per pound of lean body mass per day to ensure adequate recovery from hard training.

High quality sources of protein are those which contain all of the essential amino acids we need for repair and growth. These sources include meat, fish, dairy and eggs.

Fat

Fats, which are also known as triglycerides, are composed of fatty acids and glycerol. There are two types of essential fatty acids we need to consume in our diet: alpha linolenic acid (omega 3) and linoleic acid (omega 6).

Fats have received an undeserved bad reputation in recent years, but the truth is that we need to ingest a fair amount of healthy fats in our diet to ensure proper cell function and hormone production. This includes eating the much-maligned saturated fats as well. Fat also provides lots of energy for the body at 9 calories per gram, more than twice the caloric content of carbs.

Good sources of fat include fats from animals and fish, butter from grass-fed cows, egg yolks, avocados, coconut oil, and extra virgin olive oil. Avoid anything processed and unnatural like margarines and vegetable oils such as corn and canola oil.

The Carbohydrate Problem

Carbohydrates are the only non-essential macronutrient. When carbohydrates are ingested, the end result is glucose. Glucose enters the blood stream, where it can quickly become toxic, so the pancreas releases the storage hormone insulin to keep blood glucose levels normalized. The glucose is either used immediately for energy, shuttled into our muscle tissue or liver to be stored as glycogen, or converted to fatty acids by the liver and stored as body fat.

You can see the issue already with excess carbohydrate consumption. Once we exceed our body's glycogen storage capabilities, which is only approximately 400 grams in our muscle tissue and 100 grams in our liver, the remaining carbs are converted to stored fat.

Let me be clear, though, that excess protein and fat will also make you fat. By the same token, you can still lose body fat with carbs in your diet, so long as you have established a caloric deficit.

However, high levels of blood glucose are problematic. Chronically high blood sugar levels lead to obesity, diabetes, and chronic inflammation.

ATP is the Key

As discussed earlier, ATP is our body's energy currency; it is what fuels our muscles and our other body systems. ATP can be synthesized by the breakdown of all three macronutrients, not just carbohydrates. My point here is don't be fooled into thinking your body needs carbohydrates (glucose) to operate efficiently.

My question to those whose primary goal is improved body composition is when given the choice, why would you construct your diet around carbohydrates as the primary macronutrient? They are not specifically required by your body, and excess consumption of them leads to a myriad of health consequences. Meanwhile, people struggle to keep dietary fats to an absolute minimum when they are absolutely necessary to your health and performance.

Counting Calories

I'm not a huge proponent of solely counting calories, because fat loss is not strictly a game of calories in versus calories out.

Fat storage and fat loss is also regulated by the hormones in your body, which respond to the types of food that you eat, so food quality, food timing, and macronutrient ratio all play important roles in weight loss, as well. Because our bodies are always seeking homeostasis, our metabolisms are flexible and can adjust to short-term fluctuations in calorie intake without much issue, so simply cutting calories is just part of the picture.

I'm not suggesting that you don't need to be mindful of your calories. You can't consistently overindulge with even the most nutrient rich, whole, natural foods and not pay the price. It's always important to stay in your lane regarding your caloric intake. However, I'm suggesting that when you are consistently fully hydrated and following a diet composed of whole, natural, unprocessed foods that actually meet your nutritional needs, you can begin to listen to your body and learn to eat to satiety. Ideally, this means that you will no longer experience the impulse to eat excessively and you can trust using satiety as your guide.

Even the most complex caloric formulas only provide a ballpark figure anyway. There are just too many variables to account for, so I like to keep it super simple. I recommend starting with the following calculations. Multiply your body weight by the number 12 to determine the amount of calories you may need to hover around per day for fat loss. Multiply your body weight by 15 to determine the amount of calories you may need to hover around to maintain your weight, and multiply your body weight by 18 to determine the amount of calories you may need to hover around to gain weight.

Keep in mind that these are only ballpark figures, and calories are only part of the picture. Use this as a tool to guide you, but don't live and die by these numbers.

Ketosis and the Ketogenic Diet

Those wishing to take their low-carb eating to the extreme might want to try the ketogenic diet. The goal of a ketogenic diet, or what's commonly called a low-carb/high-fat diet (LCHF), is to enter and maintain a state of dietary ketosis. Dietary ketosis is a completely normal and natural metabolic state in which your body derives the energy it needs from ketone bodies produced in the liver from the breakdown of fatty acids. A state of ketosis is induced and maintained by eating a diet that is high in fat, moderate in protein, and extremely low in carbohydrates.

The goal is to not stimulate an insulin response in your body, as this will prevent you from enjoying the benefits of ketosis. Ingesting carbohydrates will cause a rise in blood sugar and stimulate the insulin response we don't want. Ingesting extremely high levels of protein can have the same effect.

Therefore, a ketogenic diet is not a high-protein diet. Protein is intentionally kept to a moderate level.

A general daily caloric breakdown for the ketogenic diet might consist of 80% fat, 15% protein, and 5% carbohydrates. Keep in mind that everyone is different, and some people may tolerate higher levels of protein and/or carbohydrates while still maintaining a state of ketosis.

Some people assume that ketosis is not normal, or even dangerous, because they confuse ketosis with a serious condition called "diabetic ketoacidosis," or DKA. DKA is a concern for type 1 diabetics; it is much less common in type 2 diabetics. Diabetic ketoacidosis is a condition in which both blood glucose levels and blood ketone levels are highly elevated. DKA is a serious risk for diabetics, but it is not generally a concern for healthy functioning individuals.

The purpose of pursuing a ketogenic diet is to adapt your body to efficiently utilize fat as fuel. A person who is fully adapted to a state of ketosis has literally become a fat-burning machine. In the absence of carbohydrates and the effects of the storage-hormone insulin, your body can burn stored body fat at an incredible rate.

Meal planning becomes easier on a ketogenic diet too because you've essentially eliminated one entire macronutrient from your diet. With that, your food choices become pretty cut and dried.

Most people can relate to that hungry-angry or "hangry" feeling you get when you follow a carbohydrate-based diet and it's been a little too long since you had your last meal. Eating becomes priority number one, and you can get pretty cranky in a short period of time if you're having trouble finding something to eat.

Following a ketogenic diet puts an end to that "hangry" feeling, along with the rollercoaster highs and lows that a carbohydrate diet brings to your energy levels. Increased mental clarity and consistently high energy levels are universally reported by those following the ketogenic diet.

Intermittent Fasting

Intermittent fasting is another effective strategy for boosting fat loss. Intermittent fasting is nothing more than the practice of extending your nightly fast for several hours or more to take advantage of the fat burning opportunity that fasting offers us. Fasting also condenses the window of time during which we consume our daily calories. A daily routine of intermittent fasting can be as simple as putting off your first meal of the day by just a few hours. A more aggressive approach might involve fasting 16 consecutive hours or more per day while condensing your feeding window to eight hours or less.

Intermittent fasting allows us to take advantage of longer periods of fat burning without subjecting ourselves to the restriction of calories. Fasting periods of greater than 12 hours have been shown to dramatically increase growth hormone production, which helps preserve muscle tissue and increases the use of fat storage for energy.

Intermittent fasting is much easier for people who are already following a ketogenic diet because their diet keeps them satiated, and it's much easier to go for long periods of time in between meals. In fact, it's easy to simply forget to eat because the feeling of hunger on a ketogenic diet all but disappears.

Pick Your Fuel

Carbohydrates and fats are essentially competing fuel sources. Most people do not do well eating high amounts of fat *and* high amounts of carbs; they simply get fat. On the flip side, *never* eat super low carbs and super low fats; this is a recipe for muscle loss. If you are not feeding your body the fuel it needs in the form of carbs or fats, your body will turn to its only other fuel source, amino acids It gets these amino acids from the foods you eat and by breaking down hard-earned muscle tissue!

Cheat Meals

We need to strike a balance between being strict enough to make progress and being kind to ourselves. Otherwise, we begin to resent the process.

The more consistent we can be with our eating strategy, the faster we will see progress. However, a well-planned cheat meal more or less once per week can easily be programmed into a well-designed eating strategy and provide the mental relief necessary to maintain long-term compliance to your plan.

It makes the most sense to plan your cheat meals to coincide with upcoming social events. This way you can use these events as target milestones to increase motivation and as a means to delay gratification.

Have a Meal Plan

Once you have decided on an overall eating strategy, you must have a plan. This plan must include what foods you are going to eat, in what quantities, and when. Once you know this, you can stock your fridge and prep your food in advance.

Don't approach your day relying on willpower to make healthy decisions meal to meal. Willpower is a finite resource, and it will eventually run out. You are much better off making all of the decisions regarding what to eat and when well in advance. The more you can systematize this process, the easier it will be, and the better your chances of success.

Do I Need Supplements?

The term supplements refers to a tremendously broad array of pills, potions, and powders that includes all variations and combinations of vitamins, minerals, herbs, other natural and unnatural compounds, and food-type products.

I always advise people that it's best to get all their calories and nutrients from whole food sources. Having said that, I understand that most of us do not always eat the variety of foods necessary on a weekly basis that would ensure we are getting all the vitamins and minerals we may need. Plus, who really has the time or inclination to track their intake of every single vitamin and mineral anyway? Therefore, it seems prudent to supplement with a daily multi-vitamin/ multi-mineral just to cover your bases.

When it comes to food supplements like meal replacements and protein powders, I feel these are best used primarily as a stopgap measure at times when you may not have access to quality food, or when they're needed purely as a convenience. Otherwise, you're better off planning ahead, preparing and packing your own food.

Maintain a Healthy Gut

I would be remiss if I didn't mention somewhere in this section the importance of maintaining a healthy microbiome by ensuring you are supporting a healthy gut. A detailed discussion is beyond the scope of this book, but I recommend doing your own research in this area. A healthy microbiome should naturally result from abstaining from processed foods and by eating a variety of whole, natural foods. However, for added insurance you can look into supplementing with a probiotic like *Lactobacillus*, which is also found in yogurt, sauerkraut, kimchi, and other fermented foods.

Drugs and Alcohol

We're all adults here, so just use common sense in this department. There's a time to unwind, and there's a time to get work done. If drugs and alcohol can adversely affect your judgement and behavior, then they can adversely affect your progress.

If you are following a low-carb or ketogenic diet and still intend on having a drink, then stick to clear grain alcohols mixed with club soda or diet soda. The alcohol will metabolize fairly quickly and is less likely to kick you out of ketosis.

"You don't get big and strong from lifting weights.

You get big and strong from recovering from lifting weights."

Mark Rippetoe

Chapter 4: Recovery

People tend to have a routine to their lives. They work a certain amount of hours per week, and they deal with a certain amount of work-related stress. They have relationships and other interests that create additional demands for their energy. All of these aspects of living require a certain amount of energy and produce a certain amount of stress that requires recovery. Everything we do has a price to be paid in the form of recovery.

Physical training places yet another demand on your energy resources, which is another reason why training needs to be managed and progressed at an appropriate rate so as to not overwhelm your ability to recover from the collective stressors in your life.

Training creates the stimulus for growth, but it's your ability to recover from that stimulus that allows for muscle repair, adaptation, and growth. Consistent hard training without adequate recovery is a recipe for mental and physical burnout and even injury.

Recovery is more than just allowing the soreness in your muscles to go away. Recovery also includes an appropriate period of time between intense periods of training to allow your central nervous system and other biological systems to recover, as well.

All properly designed programs will account for this need for proper recovery, and, when approached intelligently, your ability to recover will also improve over time.

Keep in mind that although your recovery ability is trainable, it also tends to decline with age. Although older trainees in their 40's, 50's and beyond are still able to tolerate high intensities (heavy weights) in their training, the volume of work they perform must be managed more closely.

There are 168 hours in the week, and even if you trained one hour every single day, that still leaves 161 hours. How you spend your time during these 161 hours away from the gym determines how well you will recover from the hard work you have invested.

The three biggest factors that govern a person's recovery are proper nutrition, which we've already discussed, quality of sleep, and overall stress reduction.

A Better Night's Sleep

Sleep is an obviously crucial recovery method, and yet many of us give very little thought to what, exactly, happens when we sleep that makes it so important. Therefore, we give very little thought to maximizing the quality of our sleep.

Life is busy, and most of us are just happy crawling into bed at the end of an exhausting day without any real thought about the process, even though we spend approximately one-third of our lives in our beds!

What Happens When We Sleep?

We fall into sleep through a series of stages from light to deep sleep. We then repeat a 90-minute cycle of alternating periods of NREM (non-rapid eye movement) and REM (Rapid Eye Movement) sleep three to six times per night.

These stages of sleep can also be defined through observed brain wave activity. Beta is our wakeful and active brain wave. Alpha is deep relaxation with eyes closed. Theta is light sleep, and Delta is the deepest and most restful sleep.

In the deepest sleep, our blood pressure lowers, our body temperature decreases, our muscles become more relaxed, tissue repair occurs, and reparative hormones such as Growth Hormone are released.

You can already see how chronic interruption of a person's sleep cycle can wreak immediate havoc on their health and well-being.

Top Sleep Strategies

Let's discuss some of the best strategies you can implement today to get a better night's sleep (in no particular order).

Early to Bed, Early to Rise

We've all heard this adage before, and it works because it aligns our own circadian rhythm to the rising and setting of the sun and the rest of the natural world around us.

If you are unable to arrange your sleep schedule in this manner, then at least establish your own consistent schedule. We are creatures of habit, and developing a consistent sleep schedule is a huge benefit to us.

Put Down Your Cell Phone

Refrain from using electronics too late in the day. The light emitted from televisions, laptops, and cell phones can suppress the body's release of melatonin and is otherwise excessively stimulating to the mind.

Say No to that Cup of Joe

You'd have to pry my morning coffee from my cold, dead

hands, but caffeine consumed too late in the day can retain its stimulating effects on the brain for many hours after consumption. That's no good for achieving the best sleep possible. This goes for any other type of stimulant, too, including nicotine. Try to avoid any consumption within six hours of bed time.

Last Call for Alcohol

Alcohol can initially help you "pass out," but in reality it has been shown to reduce Rapid Eye Movement and increase the likelihood of waking up during the night for no apparent reason.

Black It Out

Light is a powerful cue to the brain that it's time to wake up or stay awake. When it's time for bed, try to make the room as dark as possible. Eliminate all visible light from windows and doors, turn your cell phone upside down so the screen does not illuminate the room, turn your alarm clock around and throw a shirt over it, and purchase yourself a comfortable eye mask. Practice this for a while, and you'll be surprised how effective it is.

Chill Out

Your core body temperature needs to drop to initiate sleep,

so keeping the room on the cool side, below 70 degrees F, is preferable for aiding this process. The cool temperature also encourages melatonin production.

Ambient Noise

Any type of calming background noise is helpful in keeping your level of auditory stimulus fairly consistent throughout the night by smoothing over any outside sounds that may otherwise be startling or disruptive to your sleep. You don't have to get fancy here. I prefer keeping a simple oscillating fan in the room to provide white noise.

Limit Your Liquids

Limit the amount of liquids you drink later in day, especially in the several hours right before bed. All that liquid has to go somewhere, and making frequent trips to the bathroom when you could be sleeping is disruptive to both your sleep and the person you're sleeping with.

Clear Your Mind

Perform some breathing exercises, or enjoy a short period of meditation to help clear your mind before bed. Some of us may still find ourselves ruminating about the day or what tomorrow might bring. Try keeping a pen and paper next to the bed; if something truly important pops into your mind, you can write it down, let it go, and know that it can be addressed in the morning and won't be forgotten.

Stretch Out

A relaxed body is a relaxed mind, and vice versa, so spend a few minutes before or after your meditation or breathing exercises to relax into some stretching poses. Keep it light and relaxing. This isn't the time for a strenuous yoga session. Stretching allows some additional time for your mind to calm down before bed, and the added bonus will be improved mobility.

Invest Wisely

Last but certainly not least is the quality of the mattress, pillows, and bedding you sleep on. Do your research, and invest in yourself. We spend one third of our lives in bed, so it's worth it to spend what you need to get what you really want. There's a ton of options out there, so don't be afraid to experiment. Your body and mind will thank you for it.

Reduce Your Stress

Stress is a killer and a destroyer of gains. It should be obvious that anything and everything that you can do to reduce stress in your life is priority number one.

The two biggest sources of stress are work and relationships. Too many people opt for the illusion of security by staying in jobs that are neither stimulating nor fulfilling, working with or for people they don't particularly like or respect. Other people stay in toxic and abusive relationships that they know they need to leave. Both of these are silent killers and enormous sources of stress. In fact, you may have been living with elevated stress levels for so long that you no longer recognize how stressed out you really are.

If you can relate to either of these situations, then it's time to make a change. Find a new job that you actually like, and find a partner that appreciates and respects you. Everyone battles with the fear of change and of the unknown. Choose love, not fear, and watch your stress begin to melt away.

Other Recovery Strategies

There are plenty of other recovery strategies you can implement in your routine to support physical recovery and stress reduction, but make sure you've nailed down your nutrition and sleep habits and dealt with the major stressors in your life first.

Some strategies worth investigating for yourself include massage, contrast baths, cryotherapy, floatation tanks, and virtually any low-intensity physical activity.

Doing something to promote recovery is always better than doing nothing. Movement is healing, so engaging in any type of low-intensity movement that increases respiration and blood flow without contributing additional stress to your system is always better for promoting recovery than just sitting on the couch watching TV.

"If you always put limits on everything you do, physical or anything else, it will spread into your work and into your life.

There are no limits. There are only plateaus, and you must not stay there, you must go beyond them."

Bruce Lee

Chapter 5: Closing Thoughts

My sincerest hope is that this book has offered you a clearer perspective on the physical transformation process as a whole and provided some ideas and strategies that you can immediately incorporate into your own approach on your path to achieving your goals.

If I have helped even one person avoid the mistakes that I've made in my own journey so far, then I consider this project to be a huge success.

Find Your Tribe

We are social animals, and everyone learns and performs better as part of a team. That team can be big or small, near or far, physical or online, but the journey is much more enjoyable when it's shared with others. Stretch your comfort zone, and seek out others who have also committed to the same healthy lifestyle that you have. Join a gym, share your ideas, support one another, provide encouragement, and celebrate one another's achievements.

Embrace the Journey

Training is a life-long pursuit, and there are no overnight

success stories. The true goal is to continue to deepen the connection you have with your own mind and body, constantly learning what works for you and what doesn't, and adapting your training strategies over time to reflect your increasing level of knowledge and experience. Keep listening to your body, and stay flexible in your approach. Never stop exploring your limits, and never stop pushing yourself.

Enjoy The Process

At the end of the day, this process should be fun. Training and dieting and all the rest of it is hard work, but don't allow it to devolve into some type of grim duty. The pursuit of your goals should enrich your life, not take away from it. Be kind to yourself, and have fun!

"The Iron never lies to you.

You can walk outside and listen to all kinds of talk, get told that you're a god or a total bastard.

The Iron will always kick you the real deal.

The Iron is the great reference point, the all-knowing perspective giver. Always there like a beacon in the pitch black.

I have found the Iron to be my greatest friend.

It never freaks out on me, never runs.

Friends may come and go, but two hundred pounds is always two hundred pounds."

Henry Rollins

Made in the USA
Lexington, KY
27 July 2018